Life in the Cave
Overcoming Graves' Disease

LIFE in the CAVE

OVERCOMING GRAVES' DISEASE

CELIA MARIE

Celia Marie, LLC
2020

For Ri

You are everything to me and
you are God's mouthpiece in your generation.
I love you, Ri.

Joel 2:28

ACKNOWLEDGEMENTS

Pat--thank you for your financial support and for providing the much needed medical insurance. Malachi 3:10

Glynis--I could have never made it without you! Thank you for your love and for being there for my family during my surgery. Thanks for all of your prayers and the laughter! Proverbs 17:22

Pastor W. Donald and Betty Price, The Late Dr. John and Peg Howerton, Pastor Dan and Pamelia LaPaglia, Todd and Barbara Kane, Glynis Bonser, Debbie (Welch) Lowe, Richard Pollak and Garry Lowe--each of your prayers have been such a source of strength and encouragement for me and my family. I love all of you dearly and you all are like family to me. (Of course Dan and Pamelia are family!) Thank you for your belief that I would not die but live. Psalm 118:17

Eric--thank you! Jeremiah 29:11

FOREWORD

I confess to feeling apprehensive when Celia approached me about writing this entry. I immediately thought of a number of our mutual friends and acquaintances whom I believed to be more worthy and better assets to her offering. After relating this to her, Celia, in her normal grace, convinced me of the reasons that her finger pointed in my direction. So with her words clearly in my memory, I humbly pick up my pen and offer these words.

As a person who has also travelled the long road from illness to diagnosis and all of the avenues in between, I readily identified with Celia Marie's journey. In this journal of the beginning phases of a disease that has forever changed her life, Celia, exposes not only the confusion related to symptoms of early disease but has also outlined the influence of culture and spirituality upon the winding road from diagnosis to treatment...some of which kept her from seeking early assistance.

Life in the Cave is a story of Celia Marie's journey with Graves' Disease, yet, I believe that anyone who has suffered through a chronic diagnosis will be able to see the mirror of recognition turned towards them.

Celia has crafted her story with honesty, sensitivity, and humility. She has seen a need and found a way to fill it. Due to lack of informational accounts from those living with this ailment, Celia stepped into the void to offer her story...her powerful, sad, yet hopeful story. With courage and optimism, she has laid her heart before you like a living sacrifice.

Although the book that you now hold in your hands chronicles my friend's journey with Graves' Disease, if we are truly willing to reflect, I believe that like Celia Marie, we can all admit to being cave dwellers.

--Zayne Spencer
2009

INTRODUCTION

An Irish doctor, Robert James Graves, discovered Graves' Disease in the 1830s. A decade later, German doctor Karl Adolph von Basedow reported the same symptoms as Dr. Grave. Europeans are more likely to be familiar with Basedow's disease which is the same as Graves' Disease. I'm an American and, thus, will be referring to my formal diagnosis of Graves' Disease throughout my journal.

Famous celebrities and public figures who have been diagnosed with Graves' Disease include Joe Biel, George H.W. Bush, Barbara Bush, Toni Childs, Rodney Dangerfield, Bobby Engram, Marty Feldman, Diane Finley, Heino and Maggie Smith. The second president of the United States, John Adams, reportedly suffered from Graves' Disease, too.

Graves' Disease is a thyroid disorder caused by an autoimmune reaction. The trigger for the autoimmune reaction was still unknown at the time of this writing. Although Graves' Disease is not curable, it is treatable.

I was compelled to write about my personal journey with Graves' Disease because there was a lack of writings out there dealing with this unique disease. I believe that you're reading this journal because either you have been diagnosed with Graves' Disease or someone that you love/know has been diagnosed with Graves' Disease.

I want to share with you that I have written this journal in a very personal and transparent style. You will start with me before my formal diagnosis of Graves' Disease and walk with me through the first two (2) years of my battle with Graves' Disease until the night before my life would change forever. It is my deepest desire that you will receive relevant information that will encourage you and bring you hope.

CHAPTER ONE

SPRING 2005

During the spring of 2005 I began to notice that I was losing a little bit of weight. I was very pleased. I had gained about twenty pounds for the past couple of years and it was very encouraging to have my clothes fit more loosely. I was beginning to get compliments on my slimmer body. What's not to love about that?

Two weeks later I noticed that I was getting tired earlier in the day than was normal. It was approaching the end of the school year. My pre-school class was getting spring fever. I figured that my antsy students' behavior may have been the reason that I was getting tired so much earlier. I really didn't think much about it after that.

We began preparing for the Spring play and, as a result, we had to walk over to a different building than we were accustomed to for practice. The building was about an 1/8th of a mile from my classroom. By the end of the week I began having some trouble with pain in one of my legs. I figured that it would go away if I didn't put a whole lot of strain on it. The Spring play came and went but the pain in my leg remained.

It was now the last week of school which was a very busy time of the school year. The end-of-year class party required a lot of preparation because I wanted to make it special for my students. The last day of school was always so bittersweet for me. I thought that I was doing a great job keeping it hidden just how fatigued I really was and how much the pain in my leg was increasing. *Maybe all I need is a week of relaxing*, I thought.

The week between the end of the school year and the beginning of the Sizzlin' Summer school program went by way too fast. Maria (my daughter) and I looked at each other in amazement--it was now time to begin the summer program at the school.

I was so thankful to be a teacher at the school that Maria attended. It was a blessing to have her help me get my class set up for the summer session. I tried so hard to not reveal to her how tired I was and how much my leg hurt. In fact, around 1:00 p.m. each day I would experience a wave of extreme exhaustion and develop a splitting headache at that hour. I thought, *If I just take it easy this summer hopefully the fatigue and pain in my leg would subside.*

During the first month of the Sizzlin' Summer school program I began to get my edge back. I was not as tired. I was very encouraged that I had more energy. I rationalized that the less demanding schedule was the reason that I was feeling better. Really though, in the back of my mind I had not totally convinced myself that all was well. I was still losing weight and not even trying. Although very grateful for the weight loss, I couldn't help wondering if something was wrong. I thought it had to be just my imagination. Besides, Pat (my husband) seemed especially happy to have a slimmer wife by his side!

The month of June and the first part of July went by fast. It was the middle of Summer 2005 and I had lost even more weight. Now forty pounds lighter, I was excited to be able to purchase even smaller size clothes. However, the pain in my leg was getting much worse and I was limping around most of the time. I thought that I had probably just pulled a muscle because I had been exercising. I decided that it would be wise for me to lighten up on the exercising; just until my leg stopped hurting so much.

By the end of the Summer 2005 my limping was so noticeable that Pastor W. Donald Price of Cathedral Christian Center in Glendale, Arizona asked me why I was limping. I had now lost sixty pounds. Even though I was experiencing pain in my leg, I was proud to be so much thinner! My coworkers asked me if I was on a special diet and I told them, truthfully, no. I was receiving compliments all of the time on how good I looked since I had lost so much weight. I thought to myself, *I'd rather be thin even though I'm limping around.*

The Sizzlin' summer program was now over and it was the first week of August. I was participating in teacher in-service week. One of our in-service activities was a prayer walk over our campus. We would pray over each classroom. When we reached Maria's classroom, I sat down on the floor by Maria's desk. After our prayer for the students and teacher's upcoming school year, I attempted to stand up but my legs were so weak that I could not stand. I had to ask two coworkers to help me get back to my feet. Something was very wrong. I was starting to get scared. I did not know what was wrong but I did know that this was not normal for me. One of our buildings was two-story. Since I was still able to walk up and down the stairs I did not fully heed my body's warning that I needed to seek medical attention.

I stopped losing weight and the pain in my leg finally subsided. I thought that I must be getting better. The only issue that I was dealing with now was my fatigue. *Well, I am a teacher and it's the beginning of a new year*, I thought, *I must just need to give myself more time to adjust to the new school year.*

CHAPTER
TWO

FALL 2005

Because September was full of school activities and meetings I always looked forward to a break from cooking in the hot kitchen and dinner at a restaurant instead.

It is hot, I thought, *Why am I always so hot?* It was now fall and I was still hot. It felt like it was 110 degrees even though in reality, it was a comfortable seventy-four degrees inside the restaurant.

I had also discovered that whenever I went out in the sun, my eyes would literally hurt. The sun appeared so bright that I would have to squint my eyes and even entirely shut them because the sun was so painful. This is why many Graves' Disease sufferers wear dark sunglasses. That painful experience had never happened to me before. The sun was like a blinding light which hit my eyes with such force that it literally hurt.

I also noticed that my eyes were exceedingly red all of the time. I thought that they were red because I was fatigued most of the time. When you suffer from Graves' Disease you are not just a little tired. You are perpetually wiped out. You wake up tired and you are tired all of the time you are awake. It is common to experience insomnia and your eyes are prone to redness due to lack of adequate sleep.

I came to the conclusion that I was a hypochondriac. I have a Bachelor's Degree in Science with a major in psychology. I told myself that I really needed to get over this obsessive behavior and thinking about my health issues constantly.

The new school year brought a full class roster. I went home exhausted at the end of each day. I was becoming more irritable during the day. I chalked it up to being overworked. Plus, I thought that with all the new students it would probably take awhile to get into a schedule.

Maria was in third grade now and she was such a blessing as she enthusiastically helped me any way she could. We enjoyed our drive to school together and she was adjusting well to the fact that we had to come to school a half-hour earlier than her classmates because I was required to attend daily staff devotions. I was so proud of my daughter for being so mature and handling being a staff kid so well.

I used to take the stairs up to our staff devotions room daily but my legs had become so weak that I now had to take the elevator daily. This was so devastating to me because I used to enjoy walking so much. *Little did I realize that the beginning of loss that I was to experience over the next two and a half years had started in the Fall of 2005.*

CHAPTER
THREE

WINTER 2005

The first semester went by swiftly. Maria liked Mrs. Oakerman, her third grade teacher because she was consistently friendly and liked to joke with her. One day after school we went shopping for holiday outfits.

I was so very proud to be able to fit into size eight clothes again for the holiday season. I dismissed the questions that my co-workers were asking whether I was okay, and whether I thought I should see a doctor about my weight loss. In response, I thought, *No! I'm just happy to be near the weight that I used to be for so many years.*

I was getting used to the perpetual fatigue that I experienced daily. Around 1:00 p.m. each day I still became exhausted and had a splitting headache. At least after about a couple of hours the splitting headache would finally go away.

The holiday season was approaching and it was a joy to have Maria help me decorate my classroom for Christmas. We had so much fun making decorations, buying gifts for my students and creating their stockings. I love the holidays. I love the fact that secular radio stations play music about Jesus! The joy of the holiday season outweighed the concerns that I had in regards to my health issues. I chose to laugh and enjoy the holiday season with my daughter. We worked hard to prepare for my class Christmas party and it was a huge success. I was so proud of the way that Maria interacted with my students. I enjoyed serving my students during the joyous holiday season. I bought each of them a small snow globe that fit perfectly in their tiny hands.

Maria and I enjoyed our Christmas break. It was such a blessing to bake Christmas cookies and desserts together because Maria and I were always busy with all of the school-related activities most of the time. We welcomed opportunities to relax and spend part of our day doing fun activities together. On Christmas Eve day I prepared our traditional homemade lasagna (my spouse says that he married me because I bake amazing lasagna) along with Christmas Eve Cake (Torte Vigilia di Natale). Although Pat had to work on Christmas Eve and was tired while we ate our dinner we still enjoyed the tradition of our homemade lasagna dinner as opposed to going out to a restaurant. Although I was weak and had to buy pre-shredded mozzarella cheese and pre-diced onions I still boiled the lasagna pasta myself and prepared the homemade sauce. After we ate, I enjoyed playing Christmas carols and holiday music on the piano for my family. Each day was such a joy because I could relax and have fun. *I refused to dwell on how fatigued I was despite all the relaxing that I was doing--it just didn't make sense to be constantly fatigued and I just wanted to focus on the joy of the season.*

I continued to experience the splitting headaches around 1:00 p.m. each day every afternoon. Towards the end of Christmas break I became ill with walking pneumonia. It was horrible to be so ill. The antibiotics were not working and my 104 degree temperature wouldn't go away. I had to have my doctor prescribe a stronger antibiotic. I was miserable. I went to the doctor and discovered that I had walking pneumonia. He prescribed an antibiotic but after taking the full ten days prescription I was still running a high fever. He prescribed a stronger antibiotic. It isn't unusual to contract communicable illnesses when working with young children. I didn't link the walking pneumonia with the fatigue I was feeling because my doctor shared that walking pneumonia had been going around during the holidays that year.

It was now 2006 and we had a nice Valentine's Day (we called it Senior Friend Day because we honored the seniors in our families and extended family/close friends) party at the school. Once again, my daughter helped me set up my classroom for the party. We made special valentines for each student. C.J.'s (a student of mine) amazing mom, Kelly, organized the special Valentine craft projects. She was a Godsend. I always looked forward to seeing Kelly; she was so balanced and always a pleasure to interact with. Rochelle (her sweet and cheerful son Joshua was in my class) was a very supportive parent who had organized our class Harvest party during the fall semester. Glynette, my student Tiffany's mom, was quick to offer an encouraging word to me and we would often laugh together. Glynette treated me with a lot of respect and kindness; I treasured my friendship with Glynette. These are examples of a few of my very supportive parents. I thanked God for them.

SPRING 2006

I made it through the Parent Teacher conferences even though it was so exhausting preparing for them. I cannot believe that I had such a big class. I was so thankful that the Lord gave me strength to get through each day despite the ever increasing fatigue. I was also beginning to notice that I had to use the restroom more often. I thought I was just drinking too much water. Even one of my coworkers commented on how much more often I was using the restroom. We joked about it but this was just one more cause for concern that I began to ponder.

Beginning in March of 2006 I started falling asleep at work. My students would laugh and Tiffany, one of my outgoing students, would say "Teacher, wake up!" as she giggled.

I noticed that my hair was beginning to fall out. I also observed that my neck area was slightly swollen. Sandy and June, my coworkers, noticed the swelling, too. Even though I knew in my heart of hearts that something was wrong, I still was trying to dismiss all of these observances as hypochondria. In retrospect, I believe that I continually dismissed my symptoms because I was so very frightened that once I saw a doctor the diagnosis was going to be very serious. I was just not ready to emotionally deal with whatever my medical condition was.

One day my boss came into my classroom and said, "You are anxious, aren't you?" It was all starting to fall apart. I couldn't hide the symptoms any longer because they were beginning to be noticeable by others. I didn't know what to do. I loved teaching. I loved being with my students. I loved their excitement and wonder at the world they were discovering. I enjoyed having Maria come into my classroom at the end of the day. Sometimes she brought one of her friends with her.

I had been teaching since the Spring of 2000 at the school, and, as a result, my daughter and I had practically lived there for the past six years. I believe that deep down I knew that my days at the school were coming to a close. I was getting scared.

We were once again approaching the end of another school year. I was so exhausted that I was actually relieved that the school year was almost over. Maria helped me plan the end-of-year school party. I didn't do as much as I had done in the past. I was just too fatigued. I was thankful that

Kayden's (my soft-spoken student) mom, Angela, helped with the party. She was another very supportive parent.

Maria and I had our week-long break before the Sizzlin' Summer school program began. I was exhausted that whole week at home and was not physically, mentally or emotionally ready to come back for the school's summer program. By this time I could no longer hide my illness from my husband, Pat. He noticed that something was wrong. I told him that I just could no longer work at the school. He agreed. He was excited because he thought I would have time to be his loan officer for his real estate clients. *Neither one of us realized that I was only going to get much, much worse.*

On June 9, 2006 I turned in my resignation. It was one of the most painful days in my life. My friend, Carla, really helped me get through that day. I was an emotional wreck. I remember crying as I told Glynette that I was quitting. I had known Glynette for the past two years because two of her older daughters whom I dearly loved had also been in my pre-school class.

My daughter helped me pack up all of my teaching supplies. My Buick Skylark was totally full of over six years worth of teaching supplies along with gifts that I had received from students and coworkers. As we drove away with tears in our eyes we struggled to grasp the reality that we would never be coming back to Cathedral Christian Academy.

CHAPTER
FOUR

SUMMER 2006

Now that I was officially unemployed, I started sleeping later and later in the mornings. I thought I was just catching up on rest. Pat would go to work in the mornings and come home to the same dirty dishes on the dining room table that were there when he had left for work earlier that day. I was getting to the point where I just did not have the strength to do the smallest of tasks. Our home was more and more cluttered. I could not keep up with the daily chores. Pat was not only working full time along with working on real estate transactions, he was also starting to do the household chores. He didn't realize that I literally could not do the chores. I was so exhausted. I didn't have any strength. In fact I was so weak that I could no longer get up from sitting down without having to hold on to something for support.

Not only did I observe that I was sleeping more and more and becoming even weaker, I was now losing actual clumps of hair instead just strands of hair like I had in the past.

It was heartbreaking because my hair used to be so long, thick and naturally wavy. I would cry when I brushed my hair because handfuls would come out. I was so frightened.

The summer was over and it was our wedding anniversary weekend. We decided to go to Flagstaff to celebrate (Flagstaff is where we went on our honeymoon eleven years prior). While we were in Flagstaff we decided to drive up to Williams where my brother lives.

We went to visit my brother and sister-in-law during early September. My brother observed that I was very nervous, had lost a lot of hair and weight, and could barely walk--he told me to go see a doctor right away. He later shared with me that my appearance that day was such that I looked as if I had aged twenty to thirty years since he last saw me.

A few days after visiting my brother I was asked to play a grand piano at a college restaurant on an ongoing basis. I accepted the gig and didn't anticipate any problems because I had been playing the piano for thirty-eight years. One day as I began to play my set I looked at the musical notes in front of me and had no idea what they were. I was very frightened. "What is happening to me?" I asked myself. On the way home from one of my piano playing sessions, I started scratching my eyelid because my eye felt gritty. We stopped at a store and my husband noticed that my eye was all bloody on the eyeball. It also appeared that my eyes had a frightened look and were slightly protruding. It was at this point that I knew that I had to see a doctor. Pat was scared that I might have an aneurysm. I believe that it was at this point that he finally realized he had a seriously ill wife who needed medical attention immediately.

I was able to see my family doctor the very next morning. I shared with him all of my symptoms. He had his nurse immediately draw my blood. My heart rate was 125 bpm. The normal heart rate is between 60-100 bpm. My blood test results came back as critical toxic. My doctor told me that he believed I was suffering from hyperthyroidism and Graves' Disease. He prescribed Propranolol, a beta blocker which is a drug used to reduce the heart rate, and Methimazole, an anti-thyroid medication.

The function of the thyroid is to take iodine and convert it into thyroid hormones which affect nearly all tissues of the body regulating the body's metabolism. In fact, the thyroid's function is critical because it keeps the body's metabolism from over or under working.

The following morning I received a call from my doctor's office. I was to have a thyroid scan uptake within seventy-two hours and an ultrasound during the following week because he wanted to determine what the problem was with my thyroid. He didn't say what he was anticipating finding.

I was so scared. By now I needed assistance getting in and out of the car. I walked very slowly. I needed help lifting my legs from the parking lot to the actual sidewalk. I was very confused. My hands trembled so much that I could no longer write legibly. I could not focus. I was a mess. *What if I have thyroid cancer?* I thought.

CHAPTER
FIVE

During the month of October 2006, the thyroid scan and ultrasound were performed. The thyroid scan uptake was a two-day process. I was so frightened to have this test administered. I again asked myself, "what if I have thyroid cancer?" A few days after the thyroid scan uptake, I went to another center for the ultrasound. Based on the results of these tests, I was officially diagnosed with Hyperthyroidism and Graves' Disease.

I met with Dr. Richard Dolinar, my thyroid specialist, weekly. He informed me that I could no longer drive an automobile until we could get my body stabilized and my confusion subsided. I was also to refrain from exercising; it was just too dangerous to attempt to exercise in my fragile, unstable physical condition.

My heart rate was still around 130 bpm---this was an alarming rate. The threat of congestive heart failure was staring me in the face. The thought of death was very real to me. I did not want to lose my nine year old daughter. I did not want Maria to experience the loss of her mother. She was too precious to me for me to give up on life. She was my life.

During this time, I was attempting to homeschool Maria, which was a very daunting task. We were utilizing the A Beka Academy DVD curriculum (A Beka was the curriculum that my daughter studied at Cathedral Christian Academy and the curriculum that I had used with my classes). Although the lesson plans were prepared for me, it was still difficult to keep up with her lessons.

I was getting weaker and weaker. I finally had to call A Beka Academy and explain how very ill I was. I asked for an extension for my daughter because we were so behind in her schoolwork. It was granted. Praise God! I was very thankful that A Beka Academy granted the extension for Maria's schoolwork.

My eyesight was also affected. I would see ripples (like the rippling water of a stream) in front of me. It lasted for several minutes. I never knew when this would occur. It was now getting to the point where I had trouble reading.

Pat continued to work full time, work on real estate deals when he wasn't at his full time job, and keep up with the household chores. It hurt me to watch him struggle with all of these responsibilities. I could see that the strain of all of the pressure was getting to him. I felt like such a failure. I saw the fear in Maria's eyes and that hurt me so much, too. My life was becoming so painful to live. Not only was I in physical, emotional and mental pain; Maria and Pat were experiencing pain too. "Why are we going through all of this suffering?" I lamented. The hardest part was to watch their pain and to feel so hopeless and helpless in helping them heal because my illness was the source of their pain. I wanted to make their pain go away so that they could take the shackles off of them that my Graves' Disease was causing so they could be free of the "what if's"--especially for Maria. Maria and I have always been close. She is my only child. My pregnancy with Maria was high-risk; there was even a period when I was on bed rest. We are literally together 24/7. I can count on one hand the times that Maria was left with a babysitter and the babysitter was a family member.

Throughout Maria's life she has even slept with me on several occasions at night. In fact, when I first started seeing Dr. Dolinar Maria began sleeping with me again at night. We have never been self-conscious about public displays of affection. We're comfortable holding hands, kissing and embracing in front of others.

During November, I began to receive encouraging e-mails from Pastor W. Donald and Betty Price. They were my pastors for several years and have shown tremendous support and love to me and my family for over 20 years. They shared that they were taking "a stand for miracles to become evident because we are trusting and believing in (His) word." As I read their e-mail around midnight, the presence of God came into my home office in a mighty way. I responded to their email with "Yes, He is our Healer and Miracle Maker-- oh, how I believe that completely." I had also begun to read twenty-four Bible verses daily dealing specifically with healing.

During mid-November, I met with Dr. Dolinar and he informed me that it was time to schedule the Radioactive Iodine (RAI) treatment. November 19, 2006 was the day I was to go to the hospital for this treatment. A few days before the treatment I needed to begin taking steroids in an effort to keep my eyes from continuing to bulge after I stopped taking Methimazole, the anti thyroid medication.

I chose the Radioactive Iodine treatment over the Thyroidectomy option because the treatment was less invasive than surgery and I was so very frightened to go under the knife. The thought of a surgeon slitting near my vocal chords was not what I wanted to experience—I loved to sing and didn't want to have any damage done that would change or ruin my voice.

It was the evening before I was to go to the hospital for the Radioactive Iodine (RAI) treatment. I needed to make sure that I had everything ready for my return home. I was to be quarantined for awhile. I couldn't be in too close of proximity to others for a few days. I had to use special eating and drinking utensils. I had to sanitize the areas that I used before others could enter the area.

It was very difficult for me to accept that I would not be able to hug and kiss Maria for a while. We had always been affectionate with each other. I enjoy giving Maria a quick hug or kiss as a way of affirming her. I like to be physically close to her and I didn't like that opportunity to be taken away. I would never again take for granted the freedom to be physically close to Maria.

Before I went to sleep I prayed, "*Father God, please go before me. Please be with each medical staff personnel who will be part of this RAI treatment. Please let this treatment be effective and heal me of Graves' Disease and Hyperthyroidism. Please take away my daughter's, my husband's and my fear. Please help me to relax so that I can get some sleep tonight. In Jesus' name I pray, Amen.*"

CHAPTER
SIX

On the drive to the hospital I could definitely feel the prayers of intercessors for me. Their prayers helped me to stay calm and peaceful. Maria went with me to the hospital. We spent over an hour waiting to be called. Then we met with the technician. He discovered that a required blood test had not been administered. This meant that I had to go to the basement of the hospital to get my blood drawn. We then waited nearly two hours to receive the results of that required blood test. By now we had been at the hospital for nearly four (4) hours. I finally was called in for the RAI treatment. The actual treatment didn't take long at all. We all joked about how I would be glowing now that I had taken the radioactive capsules!

I was so relieved to be going home. I was so excited that this treatment was going to stop my overactive thyroid, my bulging eyes would shrink back to their normal size and I wouldn't have to take the beta blockers anymore. *I thanked God for modern medicine. It will be nice to get my energy back for the Christmas holidays*, I thought.

About a week before Christmas my whole family was ill. We went to the doctor and were all diagnosed with walking pneumonia. Since the doctor told us that it was going around I did not connect that it could be something more serious causing my immune system to be weakened. We spent Christmas at home and concentrated on healing. This was the second Christmas in a row that I had been ill with walking pneumonia. Because we were contagious we discouraged family and friends from visiting. It was a disappointment to not be able to join in on the holiday festivities. *Little did I realize at the time what a huge disappointment the RAI treatment was going to prove.*

I continued to see Dr. Dolinar monthly. The anti thyroid medication helped my body gain the weight back that I should have been at for my height and body type. I no longer had weight loss issues; in fact, I was now two dress sizes bigger much to my chagrin. My thyroid levels improved a little which was great. However, I was starting to have more complications with my eyes. Dr. Dolinar recommended that I see an ophthalmologist. Graves' Disease not only affects the eyesight but the actual structure of the eye area. It is common for the muscles around the eye to begin to swell (just like the swelling of the neck area due to the goiter--enlarged thyroid) when you have Graves' Disease.

I was still very fatigued. I now was experiencing major issues with insomnia. I also had horrible nightmares. Everything was working against me--I was afraid to go to sleep because of the nightmares but I was also so exhausted that I couldn't help but fall asleep. Then, I would wake up as soon as I reached a deeper phase of sleep due to the nightmares. It was a very frustrating and frightening cycle to go through every night.

I still experienced confusion and lack of focus. I gave up reading and watching movies because I just could not concentrate for more than a few minutes at a time. Confusion and lack of focus are common symptoms of Graves' Disease sufferers.

I had reverted back to my old ways of not revealing to my family how truly awful I felt. On December 28, 2006 my mother-in-law, Carole, had been diagnosed with Stage 4 lung cancer. A few weeks after she was officially diagnosed with cancer, I offered to help her. She was trying so hard to be brave and strong. It was a very humbling time for both of us because we were both so ill yet trying to support each other. My heart broke watching the demise of her health. I was so scared wondering what would happen if I had thyroid cancer. I saw how much pain that she was in and it frightened me so much to see such a strong and courageous woman fighting for life and losing.

I did the best that I could while taking Carole to her doctor appointments and administering her meds. This was a sobering time for us. Maria was with us while I attempted to take care of my mother-in-law. She was so scared that her grammy was going to die. I knew that she was also scared that her mommy was going to die. It hurt me to see my nine year old daughter experiencing so much stress and fear. I felt so helpless.

It was now my forty-fourth birthday. I had lost a lot of hair. I was very depressed. A young woman at church told my husband that I looked "scary". Her comment really hurt me because I used to be attractive. I just wanted to die. Then I remembered my beautiful daughter, Maria, and I thought of the times in my life when I had to make the choice to live. When I was born the doctors told my parents that I had cerebral palsy, one of my legs was shorter than the other which would cause me to walk with a noticeable limp, and my eyesight was so damaged that I would eventually become blind. I proved the doctors wrong and never grew into any of those 'labels'. My parents provided the best care for me and through corrective eye surgery and several years of concentrated eye care I no longer needed to wear glasses.

Years later as an adult, once again I was faced with the choice to live. I wanted to see Maria grow up. I wanted to be at her high school graduation. I wanted to see her walk down the aisle on her wedding day. I wanted to share my life with her future children and enjoy watching them grow up. Now that I was a mom I chose desperately to live to watch my daughter "become." I wanted to share my thoughts with her on the choice to live and see if she had similar beliefs or if she would carve her own way. Choosing to live is one of the bravest choices one can ever make. I could not allow myself to give up on life even though, at that moment, I was just so exhausted and so broken; I was broken physically, emotionally, mentally, and spiritually. At this point, I stopped reading the twenty-four healing verses daily. I stopped going to church. I didn't even feel like praying anymore. In retrospect, I believe it was at this breaking point I subconsciously chose to live even though I halted my spiritual nourishment.

I remember the fear in Maria's eyes as we celebrated my birthday. I told her that everything would be okay. I assured her that I was not doing to die. We hugged and cried together. Knowing that Maria was suffering and fearful made me angry. As a mom, I wanted to protect her from all the bad of the world. I was a complete failure. I felt so sorry for my husband. The attractive woman that he married years earlier was gone. I was even ugly on the inside. I had lost hope. I began to believe that I wasn't going to be healed. I felt so lost.

It was during this winter season that I began to experience the first stirrings of what I would later refer to as life in the cave. I was aware that life was going on around me but for me time stood still. I was trapped in the prison of disease watching others (they were like shadows) going about their lives. They were going to work, going to the grocery store, going to church and going to the movies as I sat chained and motionless. I could see the light of life in a very far distance but directly all around me was darkness. I saw the outline of steps leading to a tall, locked gate far off in front of me and beyond that gate there were steps leading higher to the light. I often wondered if I would ever make it to the light and beyond.

CHAPTER
SEVEN

Carole was getting worse. The family called in a formal nurse to take care of her. I was relieved because I was in no shape to take care of her; plus, Maria was negatively affected by being around seriously ill loved ones. Maria was sad and scared most of the time and she would often cry. She would tell me that she didn't want me to die and hold on to me for dear life.

Although this winter season had begun to descend upon me, I still was reaching out to a friend of a friend. I had learned (while reading a post on the 77s, a Sacramento-based band, listserv) that Jan Volz was requesting prayer for Eric (his son) because he had been wrongfully accused of murder. In 2000, I had formed a prayer group and I asked my prayer group to pray for Jan's son, Eric. Jan added me to his master e-mail group and faithfully gave updates on Eric's situation. Eric had been falsely accused of murdering his ex-girlfriend, Doris Jimenez, on November 21, 2006 and he was still sitting in a jail in Nicaragua more than a month after his arrest. Eric's family was doing everything possible to get him back to the United States but the Nicaraguan authorities refused to release Eric. Not only was I scared for Carole's losing battle with cancer and my possible prognosis of thyroid cancer--I was also very scared for Eric. I had no idea, at the time, that it would take approximately another year for Eric to be released from prison.

On February 21, 2007 Eric Volz was sentenced to thirty years in prison--Nicaragua's maximum sentence. Eric, falsely accused, was suffering the gravest of injustices and inhumane treatment. This totally devastated me to know how much pain Eric, his dad, his mom, his sister and loved ones were experiencing. My family had gone through a similar situation six years earlier, thus, I had so much empathy for the Volz and Anthony families. Eric's horrific situation was the catalyst for me to begin praying again. Another reason Eric's story caught my attention was because since I was a child I wanted to drive on the Pan American Highway through Nicaragua, Costa Rica and on to see the Panama Canal. To learn that Eric was being tortured in Nicaragua touched a personal chord of interest. I knew that the only way that I could help the Volz and Anthony families was to pray. Even though I did not believe in a miracle for myself I knew that God could open those prison doors for Eric just like He had for Paul and Silas. I was very uninhibited in my prayers for Eric's freedom. I was also praying for Doris' family and specifically for justice for Doris and that her true murderers would be revealed and apprehended. The prayers were also being lifted up for Maria. As the days turned into weeks and then into months I discovered that I was actively involved in daily prayer again.

Two days after Eric's sentencing, on February 23, 2007 Carole lost her battle with lung cancer. I wrote this to my prayer group: "This morning as I held Carole's hand she began to cross over the Jordan River--at approximately 11:40 a.m. she made it to the other side." I truly loved her. Not only had I lost my mother-in-law, I had lost my sister in the Lord. I would never hear her say "God bless" nor "how's my Celia?" and I would never experience the warmth of her hugs again. *Carole's death would officially begin my experience with life in the cave for the next eighteen months.*

CHAPTER
EIGHT

SPRING 2007

Today, March 13, was my daughter's tenth birthday. We had a pizza party and celebrated with a Carvel cake. I enjoyed watching Maria laugh and play with her best friend Tabitha on her special day. For the last nine months Maria had worn such a sorrowful countenance and it warmed my heart to see her smile, giggle and chuckle for hours that day with Tabitha.

The day after her birthday, Maria was crying. I asked her what was wrong and she replied, "I miss Grammy. I wish that Grammy could have been here for my birthday." I knew my daughter was missing the special tradition she normally shared with her grandmother. They would spend time together, just them, usually going to lunch and then to Toys R Us. I knew that this had been terribly special to Maria, and now all I could do was give her a big hug and hold her until her sobs subsided.

About a week after her birthday, my husband took Maria and Tabitha to the humane society. They fell in love with an Australian Cattle Dog, christened Boomer at the humane society, and brought him home. Boomer was a wonderful new addition to the family. He was so well-behaved and very gentle. Boomer was tri-colored with the majority of his body black. His face looks like a beagle's and he has a white Bentley stripe above his nose. His black tail has a white tip. Boomer never jumped on a person and he never begged for food. The moment I looked into Boomer's beautiful brown eyes I fell in love with him. That night he chose to sleep right beside me on the floor and he still sleeps right beside me on his very own leather bed!

A few days after Boomer came to live with us we noticed that he had nightmares. We would gently wake him up and reassure him that he was okay, we loved him and would not hurt him. We would tell him that he was safe now.

Boomer often experienced his nightmares at the same times I was up with anxiety attacks. We were some pair. I finally just had to keep the TV on a Christian TV station all night long so that when I woke up with an anxiety attack I could calm myself down more easily. Once I awoke I rarely ever went back to sleep.

Due to the lack of sleep, I was also extremely irritable all of the time which put an incredible strain on my family. Further, Dr. Dolinar shared with us that it is common for several married Graves' Disease sufferers to divorce because the personality of the Graves' Disease sufferer tremendously alters and perpetual irritability is a common symptom. In fact in some marriages it is too difficult for the healthy partner to adjust to the personality (emotional and mental) changes that occur in the Graves' Disease sufferer.

Pat continued to work long hours through the month of June while Maria and I daily conducted open houses at a property Pat had listed. Meanwhile, our house remained cluttered and the daily tasks continued to exhaust me. I was becoming more and more anxious as each day seemed to drag on with more clutter, more fatigue and more financial stress.

Dr. Dolinar checked my blood levels and discovered that my thyroid levels were sky-high again when I saw him in June for my regular three-month appointment. My pulse was also rapid. He prescribed Methimazole once again. I didn't like taking the Methimazole because it made me gain weight but I noticed I wasn't as anxious when I took the Methimazole so I began taking it again. He also increased my dosage of

Propranolol, the beta blocker. He told me that if I continued to feel anxious he would prescribe an anti-anxiety med for me.

My husband was planning a trip to Bushnell, Illinois for the annual Cornerstone Music Festival during the last days of June and first days of July. He hadn't been able to attend for several years and he wanted to take us for a family vacation along with his best friend's family of six. I did not want to go to Cornerstone because I was still feeling weak, confused, fatigued and anxious. Dr. Dolinar advised me not to go. I explained to him that this was a very special event that Pat rarely attended so Dr. Dolinar prescribed an anti-anxiety med and told me to call him any time on the trip if I needed to talk to him. *I never took the anti-anxiety med because I was too scared of the side effects that it could have on me.*

CHAPTER
NINE

SUMMER 2007

On the last Sunday of June 2007 we all loaded up in the RV and headed out for Cornerstone. We had six blowouts before we ever made it out of our home state. I was already a nervous wreck but I told Pat that I would go with him if he really wanted me to, so it was now Cornerstone or Bust!

We stayed at KOA Kampgrounds. I had never been RVing in my life. If I hadn't been so ill, I believe that I really would have enjoyed the experience more. We were supposed to arrive at Cornerstone on Wednesday morning but because of the issues with the tires we wound up arriving during the late afternoon on Thursday. I was already very irritated because I missed several of the bands that I wanted to see. I remember changing clothes in the RV and rushing (as best as I could because I was still very weak) to see Leigh Nash of Sixpence None the Richer. I got there just in time to hear her sing two songs before the end of her set.

Because I was so weak, Pat rented a golf cart for us so that we could get around the huge festival grounds. I spent each day at the Gallery Tent. There were a few bands playing there that I liked. I was content although my perpetual exhaustion put a damper on my happiness.

Sunday morning came way too fast and it was time to leave. Literally minutes before we left Cornerstone, Zayne (an internet friend whom I had never personally met) knocked on our RV door. Zayne told me that she vowed she wasn't going to leave Cornerstone until we finally got to meet in person. It was such a joy to spend about twenty minutes visiting with

Zayne. We had been internet friends for about three years when we connected on the 77s listserv. We were fans of other musical artists and bands, too. Over the years we shared bits and pieces of our lives through e-mail and discovered that we are both cat lovers.

After our visit we started down that dusty Cornerstone road to return home. It took us three days to drive back to Arizona. I was exhausted and so grateful to be home again. We had really missed our pets because Cornerstone wouldn't allow us to bring our pets. We arrived home on the fourth of July and I was exceedingly exhausted because we had been on the road in the RV for three consecutive days. When we walked in the house I was relieved and immediately stressed due to the total chaos of cluttering the house with two weeks of dirty laundry, bedding and camping equipment which were literally dumped in the living room, dining room and kitchen area. My husband took Maria to see the fireworks with friends so that she wouldn't miss out on the holiday festivities. After they left I went to bed totally exhausted and exasperated because of the clutter.

During the remainder of the summer I continued to have regularly scheduled appointments with Dr. Dolinar. He would measure my goiter and my eyes to see how far they had protruded in comparison with the previous visit. There was no change in the measurements. I was still struggling with anxiety attacks but they weren't as frequent as they had been in the past.

I was starting to feel a little normal in that I wasn't as tired and anxious and had even lost a couple of pounds. Dr. Dolinar reduced the dosage of my meds. My levels seemed to be holding on their own. It looked like the RAI treatment had finally taken.

I saw Dr. Dolinar in September of 2007 and he said that he wanted to see me again in December. I believe that I was still in denial during this time period. I had convinced myself that the goiter was shrinking and that my eyes weren't protruding as much. I was expecting to be told that he wouldn't want to see me for at least six months when I saw him in December. *I had no idea just how wrong I was.*

In November, Maria and I began making plans for our Thanksgiving meal. We decided that we wanted to spend Thanksgiving at a KOA Kampground. Maria and Pat worked very hard to get everything together for our Thanksgiving excursion.

Our neighbors at the KOA were from Australia. They had two teenage sons. We loved their Aussie accents. Our dog, Boomer, loved the extra attention from our neighbors. The weather was very pleasant and we had an enjoyable time on our Thanksgiving holiday. I enjoyed Maria and Pat tell of the fun experiences they had while riding in the go-cart on the hiking and go-cart trails. Boomer stayed at the campsite with me and we rested. After we rested I took him for a little walk around the KOA Kampground and up a small hiking trail.

Maria and Pat bought our Christmas tree during Thanksgiving weekend. They chose a big, beautiful fragrant Christmas tree. We were all so excited this holiday season. Our home was filled with the delicious aromas and scents of the seasons that resulted from our holiday baking. We were all extremely excited about it being Boomer's first Christmas. He appeared to sense the joy and wonder of the season, too. We had noticed that he wasn't having as many nightmares as he used to. Boomer was finally settling in. He was even gaining weight and I was gaining weight right along with him.

I went in for my December thyroid appointment. The appointment didn't last too long. Dr. Dolinar told me he wanted me to get my blood drawn that day. He said that there was no change in the measurement of my goiter and eyes. Dr. Dolinar informed me that he would call me with the results of my blood test. We wished each other a happy holiday season. I was certain that the next time I would see him again would probably be in around four to six months. *Little did I know that I would never see him again.*

CHAPTER TEN

EARLY WINTER 2007

The phone rang and Dr. Dolinar's voice came on the answering machine. I walked over to pick up the phone. He told me the results of my blood tests. He went on to say that he could no longer help me. He referred me to his colleague, Dr. Daniel Duick, who handled the "tough" thyroid cases. I started to cry and thanked Dr. Dolinar for all that he had done for me. Once again I was scared. I was going to have to start all over again. I worried about whether I would like my new specialist, and whether I would be able to trust him with my life.

It was now Christmas Eve and I prepared my annual lasagna along with the Christmas Eve Cake (Torte Vigilia di Natale). On Christmas day we had Dijon Maple Spiral Sliced Ham with all of the holiday sides and pies for dessert. My family had been enjoying this Christmas meal for a few years and I didn't want them to miss out just because I was weak. The dinner was strained because I was exhausted, Pat was stressing out about finances and Maria was hurt that we were not having a festive atmosphere at the holiday table.

On January 7, 2008 I met with my new thyroid specialist, Dr. Daniel Duick. He was very thorough; he personally performed my ultrasound. I was immediately impressed with him. He told me that he wanted to meet with me the following week to discuss our plan of action. When Dr. Duick and I met he informed me that I needed a total thyroidectomy because my goiter was huge and toxic. He said that he was surprised that I had lasted as long as I had. I was in very bad shape and was only going to get worse unless I got that toxic goiter removed from my body. He referred me to a surgeon: Dr. Richard Harding. I agreed to the surgery but I was terrified to go under the knife.

The following week I met with the surgeons, Dr. Harding and Dr. Bryce. They were young men; I had to choose whether I trusted them with my life. As my daughter and I drove away from their office, she started to cry. Maria said "Mommy, I don't want you to die." I told her that Dr. Harding and Dr. Bryce were excellent surgeons and they were going to help me get well. It was at that point that I chose to believe that I was in good hands.

My total thyroidectomy was scheduled for February 25, 2008. I had chosen the surgery to take place at a hospital very near my home.

Each day was very hectic as I tried to get everything in order for my surgery. There were a million little things to do that were all important. I was still very frightened to go under the knife. I had requested that several people, in addition to my prayer group, pray for me. An internet friend who became a great source of encouragement during this time was Marti. She was a diligent prayer warrior for myself and my family. Thank you, Marti!

I was having trouble sleeping at night because I was so frightened that I was going to die during the surgery. I tried to calm down. At times I actually did calm down for the sake of Maria because she was so frightened. I believe that the prayers that were being offered up for my family helped calm us. Many times we could sense the presence of the Lord with us.

On February 14 my daughter and my spouse brought home a beautiful, young bunny rabbit. I was very upset and irritable that they brought home a new pet so close to my surgery date; I didn't want to take the time to care for a new pet while trying to get ready for my upcoming surgery. I had to admit, though, that the bunny was adorable. It took a while for Maria to name her bunny. She finally decided to call him Snickers. Snickers enchanted us all with his winning ways. He became the perfect pet. Although Snickers could not verbally communicate, he was a very effective non-verbal communicator. He would hop excitedly to the refrigerator when I opened the door to give him a carrot, lettuce or a strawberry. Then he would perform a bunny spin in jubilation of his edible treat. He would also eagerly wiggle his nose in anticipation of his favorite foods. He was so adorable when he did his flopsies. As he grew older his markings turned sable and his fur was very soft. He was also quite curious. He thought that the telephone, computer, stereo and television cables and wires were roots. Although Snickers was just a small bunny, he brought so much light into my dark days. *At the time, I did not realize how therapeutic Snickers was going to be for me during the next nine months.*

It was now eleven days before my surgery and I still hadn't drawn up a will. I needed to make sure there were funds in the bank account to cover my insurance co-pay for the surgery. I was dragging my feet. I was scared. My friend, Glynis, (we'd been close friends for 21 years) and I were e-mailing each other. I confided to her how frightened I was. She told me that she was praying for me. A few days later Glynis said that she was going to come out to be with me the weekend before my surgery up through the day after my surgery. I was so relieved that she was coming out. Maria loved her and I knew that she would feel safe with her.

On the Friday before my surgery I finally had my will notarized and had the funds transferred into the bank account to pay for my surgery's insurance co-pay. Glynis was coming into town later on that afternoon. Everything was going as planned. She came over on Saturday and we visited, laughed, cried and prayed together.

On Sunday, the day before my total thyroidectomy, Maria and I laughed and hugged throughout the day. I told her many times that day how much I loved her. I tried my best to hide from her how frightened I was to go under the knife. God really gave me peace that day before my surgery. The day was coming to an end. Before I went to sleep I prayed, *"Father God, please help me to sleep well tonight. Please go before me for tomorrow's surgery. Guide my surgeons' hands. Let it be a successful surgery. Please let me survive so that I can watch my daughter grow up. In Jesus name, Amen."*

As I sat in the utter darkness of despair the dazzling light of hope and life became brighter. The life that I was choosing would be different than what I was accustomed to but I wanted to choose life and live my life to the fullest. I decided that I would not let my fear of Graves' Disease hold me in darkness any longer. I refused to let Graves' Disease rob me of a life filled with my daughter's beauty and the beauty of a life chosen to live in wonder of each new day.

I invite you to continue with me on my journey of living with Graves' Disease in my next book which begins in the early morning of the day of my total thyroidectomy. You will experience my memories of the first moments I woke up from surgery and the disappointments and joys of the miraculous outcome of my surgery.